THE AXEMAN

THE BRUTAL HISTORY OF THE AXEMAN OF NEW ORLEANS

COLD CASE CRIME SERIES #4

WALLACE EDWARDS

Absolute Crime Press
ANAHEIM, CALIFORNIA

ABSO|UTE CR|ME

www.AbsoluteCrime.com

Contents

About Absolute Crime..7

Introduction..*10*

Chapter 1: The Murders of a Killer with Supernatural Means...*14*

A Slaying of Alarming Brutality.................................... 16

A Second Grocer Attacked... 20

A Pregnant Woman Bludgeoned; An Elderly Barber Hacked.. 21

Chapter 2: The Killer Moves on Grocers in Gretna *25*

The City Starts to Panic.. 27

The Axeman Returns from Tartarus 30

The Axeman Visits the Boca Household..................... 31

The Final Victim: Mike Pepitone, Grocer in the Quarter 33

Chapter 3: A Suspect List as Deep as the Mississippi – On the Killer's Trail............................*36*

Clues and Leads in the Maggio Killings..................... 37

The Davi, Crutti and Rossetti Cases Collide.............. 40

The Web of Evidence Connects Known Mafiosi 41

Chapter 4: The Police Tackle the Besumer Murder *48*

Mrs. Schneider, Sarah Laumann and a Copycat on the Scene 50

Romano, Cortimiglia and Boca Fall; the System Returns 51

Chapter 5: The Apparent End to the Murders – and a Clue from California *57*

Where the Pepitone and Mumfre Stories Intersect.. 59

The Deeper, Darker Past in the Big Easy 61

Chapter 6: Four Names, One Criminal – The Elusive Monfre-Mumphrey-Mumfre-Manfre *66*

The Strings Mafiosi Played Inside the Pen and Out . 69

Chapter 7: Omerta in the Big Easy – How a Vow of Silence Kept Killers in the Shadows *74*

The Final Showdown: Where Omerta Failed and Order Was Restored 76

While One Killer Exits, Others Fade Away 82

Bibliography *84*

Ready for More? *86*

Newsletter Offer *94*

ABOUT ABSOLUTE CRIME

Absolute Crime publishes only the best true crime literature. Our focus is on the crimes that you've probably never heard of, but you are fascinated to read more about. With each engaging and gripping story, we try to let readers relive moments in history that some people have tried to forget.

Remember, our books are not meant for the faint at heart. We don't hold back--if a crime is bloody, we let the words splatter across the page so you can experience the crime in the most horrifying way!

If you enjoy this book, please visit our homepage (www.AbsoluteCrime.com) to see other books we offer; if you have any feedback, we'd love to hear from you!

Sign up for our mailing list, and we'll send you out a free true crime book!

http://www.absolutecrime.com/newsletter

INTRODUCTION

While jazz was making New Orleans buzz in the early 1900s, a vicious axe murderer almost stopped the party, igniting enough terror to evoke comparisons to London's Jack the Ripper. Neither women nor children were spared, as the killer sent taunting letters to the newspapers and mangled bodies to the morgue.

By 1919, few people felt safe at night in New Orleans. The Axeman's blade and the Mafia's Black Hand seemed to work in harmony, as locals huddled in fear and murder after murder went unsolved. The city would regain its composure in time for the Jazz Age, but the identity of the killer eluded investigators in every branch of law enforcement.

CHAPTER 1: THE MURDERS OF A KILLER WITH SUPERNATURAL MEANS

Turn-of-the-twentieth-century New Orleans was exploding with jazz music and a riot of conflicting cultures. Free blacks joined the ranks of the city's bubbling population, while Italian immigrants settled in increasing numbers from 1890-1920, representing a shift from the mainly Francophile culture of the Crescent City's past.

By the 1910s, the famed French Quarter was at least 80 percent Italian, the majority of whom were natives of Sicily, whose cooking and St. Joseph's Day rites filled city streets. As much as Sicilians brought with them a culture dating back to Ancient Greece, they also brought more recent innovations, including the Cosa Nostra.

A menacing product of the old country, the Cosa Nostra in New Orleans was its most intimidating as the Black Hand, an arm specializing in blackmail and extortion. The Hand, as it was called, targeted enterprising Italians looking to run small businesses without interference. Following the lynching of Italians in 1890 and a race riot in 1900, there was good reason to doubt the stability of New Orleans. Yet more often than not, Italians would come to fear the Mafia itself rather than seek its protection.

Upon the arrival of the Axeman of New Orleans, the city was fully enmeshed in its superstitious ways. Voodoo rites and ravenous cults were blamed for axe murders the preceding years in Louisiana, reminding residents that the supernatural demanded their respect. New Orleanians became terrified of the landscape itself, whether it was the flu epidemic brought to ports in 1918 or the bombings that rocked the Italian community for years. Whoever struck the blows attributed to the Axeman of New Orleans preyed on these fears, possibly hiding behind a Mafia mask. In any case, the killer started out with a headline murder.

A Slaying of Alarming Brutality

On May 23, 1918, New Orleans woke up to the story of a gruesome axe murder. Joseph and Catherine Maggio were hacked to death as they slept in rooms adjacent to their grocery on Magnolia Street, about midway between Napoleon and Jefferson Avenues, south of Claiborne. The story in the Times-Picayune was accompanied by photos of the dead couple inside their humble chambers. Neither money nor valuables were taken from the scene. Theft was clearly not the purpose. Murder was.

Maggio's two young brothers, arriving home from a drinking spree just after the killer struck, were arrested and charged with the crime. The police were baffled and tried to identify the clothing covered in blood (it belonged to the murdered couple). Fingerprinting was possible in 1918, but the police had yet to put the technique to work for them in any useful way. The axe found on the scene was only confiscated as evidence of how the couple was killed. The idea of connecting the axe to a killer through a scientific process was never considered. Instead, the police wandered through the neighborhood, asking questions and searching for a motive. They found more than they could have hoped for just a short walk from the crime scene. Scrawled in chalk, in the hand of a child, a message covered the asphalt:

"Mrs. Maggio will sit up tonight, just like Mrs. Toney."

It was said to be a child's handwriting, and it certainly represented the careless execution of an amateur. Speculation as to its meaning and origin abounded. Was the killer tipped off by an accomplice who knew the Maggios? It told an eerie tale, one of death messengers waiting in the night, pointing the finger to a killing about to happen. Whether it was a warning or an attempt to dissuade the killer from moving on the Maggio family that night, the message was not heeded.

Mrs. Toney's identity was also unknown, but the attention to women suggested to observers a connection to classic Mafia practices. Criminal experts past and present have understood Italian gang activities to be respectful of women and children, often sparing them, though proof in connection with New Orleans in 1918 is unconvincing. From child kidnappings to bombings of populous neighborhoods, New Orleans mobsters did not follow any type of consistent rulebook. Instead, it appears a concerted effort was made to prepare the killer for what he was to find inside the Maggio home – whether to prepare to kill a single human, or several.

What the police found at the crime scene included an axe, a razor blade, two mutilated bodies, a wooden chisel and a door panel that had been removed to gain access to the Maggio home. The axe was thought to be Maggio's own. The killer had possibly been bold enough to enter the home unarmed – through the space created by the door panel – and look through the home for a weapon. Such a tactic suggested that the killer knew where to find the axe. A great deal attention was paid to the razor used to slit the throat of Catherine Maggio, who was nearly decapitated when discovered. Police ascertained the razor belonged to Andrew Maggio, the brother of Joseph, who worked as a barber and said he'd taken it home for sharpening.

Andrew Maggio panicked. His brother and sister in law were discovered mutilated in their bed. He and his brother Jake had come home knowing nothing of the events. Later, as his memory tried to piece together moments of the drunken spree, the police confronted him with a razor and demanded to know why he'd killed the couple with it. Andrew answered unsteadily and entered police headquarters as the chief murder suspect. Once Andrew's nerves calmed, his story started to make sense. The police held him in jail during the Maggios' funeral and he never saw them again. Stinging with the embarrassment, the police released him in the following days. It was the first of many miscues made by detectives in the Axeman killings.

A Second Grocer Attacked

The following month, a second New Orleans couple was visited by the Axeman, this time across town in the city's Seventh Ward. The victims were Louis Besumer and Anna Lowe – a grocer and his common-law wife. John Zanca, a baker who made regular deliveries to Besumer's store, discovered the couple in the aftermath of the attack.

It was the night of June 28, 1918. Zanca noticed a door panel missing upon his arrival and spent several minutes knocking and shouting to make contact with Besumer. Finally he answered the door with blood dripping from his skull. Zanca called an ambulance and remained at the scene as police came to investigate. Both Besumer and Lowe survived their bout with the Axeman, though both suffered lasting damages. Lowe died in a New Orleans hospital in early August 1918.

Before passing, she fingered Besumer as the attacker. Besumer would spend several months in jail following the accusations. New Orleans police were among the few who believed Besumer was responsible for her death.

A Pregnant Woman Bludgeoned; An Elderly Barber Hacked

If a killer commits a series of murders, the perpetrator will often leave a sign of his or her presence as a trademark. Serial killers feed off of an inflated sense of self-worth deriving from these signatures. The feeling becomes magnified as the police and media publicize the details of each murder and point out the unifying elements. To believe a killing is anything other than isolated or random, this type of connection must exist.

In the next axe attack of New Orleans, whatever chain had existed was broken. A pregnant woman named Schneider awoke from her sleep to see an axe coming down on her head. It was August 5, 1918. Schneider and her husband, a local businessman, were expecting their first child within weeks. When her husband arrived home, he found the woman close to death and rushed her to the hospital. She remembered little of use to the police and told a simple tale of being struck and left to die. Somehow, Mrs. Schneider and her unborn child survived. She gave birth to a girl a few weeks later. Police found no chisel, no door panel removed and no man on the premises. Mr. Schneider, for his part, had no interest in the grocery business. The Axeman had acted on pure bloodlust.

Just five days later, New Orleans received news of another killing. Joseph Romano, an Italian barber, took the brunt of the Axeman's weapon this time. Yet there were witnesses who saw the attacker. Romano's nieces encountered a large figure dressed in black as he fled the premises. Moving gracefully and fleet of foot, he exited without considering an attack on the young women. Romano was taken to a hospital and died two days later. Police did discover a panel chiseled from the Romano home's door, identifying one telltale sign. The trademark was in place. The killer was not hiding his modus operandi, as both weapon and entry method were consistent. And once again there was no robbery, no sign of valuables disturbed. It was clear the multiple homicides were related, but speculations proved to be fruitless, as did the continued investigation by New Orleans detectives.

CHAPTER 2: THE KILLER MOVES ON GROCERS IN GRETNA

On the axe murder front, 1918 ended peacefully. World War I came to a close overseas, as Armistice was declared and victory was celebrated in the West. However, an influenza epidemic terrorized the city that winter, claiming more than 3,500 lives before it had run its course. As the flu became controlled in time for spring, the killer resumed his assaults in early 1919, this time across the Mississippi River in Gretna, Louisiana.

On the night of March 10, a commotion was heard at the home of Charles Cortimiglia and his family. Iorlando Jordano, an Italian grocer and a neighbor of Cortimiglia, arrived to discover an impossibly gruesome scene. Cortimiglia, his wife and their young baby had all been bludgeoned by the Axeman. The baby died instantly; Charles lay dying on the ground; and Rose struggled to survive a skull facture. Cortimiglia and his wife lived after being treated in a local hospital. It appeared to be another case of a madman on the loose, but Mrs. Cortimiglia held her neighbors, the Jordanos, responsible for the attack (Frank Jordano lived with his father Iorlando, an elderly grocer).

Police moved swiftly based on Rose Cortimiglia's accusation, while Charles Cortimiglia disputed his wife's claims of involvement by the Jordanos. There was a history of competition between the families, but otherwise little evidence for investigators to use. The killing of the Cortimiglia baby created a new level of hysteria in the city. An axe murderer who would not spare the life of an innocent child provoked terror all over a city where superstitious natures needed little provocation. The telltale signs were once again present: at the Cortimiglia home, a door panel had been chiseled out; an axe had been used; and no valuables or cash were stolen. The killer once again simply wanted blood.

The City Starts to Panic

As New Orleans detectives remained stumped, daily newspapers fanned the flames of hysteria by reporting Axeman sightings all across the city. Door panels removed with a wooden chisel were discovered nightly in the French Quarter and other neighborhoods. Citizens armed themselves to confront the killer. Some reported firing at the first sign of an intruder at the door. Police could not respond to even half the sightings. If every story of an axe-wielding maniac was believed, dozens of men were stalking the city, hoping for a chance to split the skulls of the innocent.

Perhaps the most famous – and maybe irresponsible – move of the period was the Times-Picayune's printing of a letter signed "the Axeman" on March 13, 1919. With "Hell" as the return address and warnings of future murders stocking every paragraph, the letter is a combination of whimsy and bloodthirsty psychosis. He taunts the police, whose efforts he says "not only amuse me, but His Satanic Majesty, Franz Josef." The killer continued his harangue on the NOPD, but hinted they actually weren't interested in catching him. "I feel sure the police will always dodge me." Yet one final, outlandish claim practically forced newspaper editors to publish the letter. Claiming to be a big fan of jazz, the killer gave the city a choice:

> *Next Tuesday night, I am going to pass over New Orleans... I am very fond of jazz music, and I swear...that every person shall be spared [where] a jazz band is in full swing...One thing is certain and that is some of your people who do not jazz it on Tuesday night (if there be any) will get the axe.*

With that, the Axeman signed off and ostensibly returned to "Tartarus." The writer's referencing Tuesday night is significant. The Feast of St. Joseph, a highly celebrated day for New Orleans residents, fell on the Tuesday in question, March 19, 1919. St. Joseph's Day meant major parties throughout the city, as it still does in New Orleans. Among Italian-Americans, estimated to represent one-third of the New Orleans population in 1919, the day was especially important.

Everyone geared up for a party that Tuesday, hoping to ward off the killer through song and celebration. Indeed, no murders were committed the night of March 19, which was said to be the most raucous night of partying in New Orleans history. In fact, one local songwriter seized the opportunity and penned a song in honor of the occasion. Titled "The Mysterious Axman's Jazz (Don't Scare Me, Papa)," the song filled the air of Crescent City homes the night of St. Joseph's Feast, amusing all who believed they were choosing the festivities over certain death. Author Joseph John Da Villa might not have had the talent of Irving Berlin, but this tune was an instant success.

For a writer whose best-known hit was "Give Me Back My Husband, You've Had Him Long E'Nuff," it is easy to speculate what a struggling songwriter could do with a pen and the address of the local newspapers. Da Villa was never accused of any such act, yet the alternative is equally troubling. A killer was on the loose. Could this vicious individual be the same one telling locals to "jazz it" or die? Whoever was behind the letter declined to give New Orleans a second chance. He waited until summer.

The Axeman Returns from Tartarus

Reports of the Axeman's next attack filled the newspapers on Monday, August 4. On early Sunday morning before dawn, a man armed with a blunt object visited the home of Sarah Laumann, an eighteen-year-old woman living in a room next door to her parents. He beat Laumann and knocked out several of her teeth, though her screams scared off the assailant before he could finish the job. Laumann's profile did not match the Axeman's previous victims, yet police located an axe outside her home and relayed the information to the press. The Axeman was back.

Almost every detail of the crime failed to jibe with other accounts. The perpetrator, instead of chiseling out a door panel, climbed into Laumann's home through an open window. Reports indicate she lost several teeth, possibly from a direct blow to the mouth, in an attempt to disfigure her rather than kill her. Detectives surmised that, if the attacker held Laumann's face down on the bed, he could have knocked out teeth with a blow to the head. Otherwise, it would suggest a point-blank assault with an object other than an axe. Laumann's attending physician told reporters the next day that it was unlikely an axe caused her injuries. Nonetheless, the story ran in every newspaper.

The Axeman Visits the Boca Household

The killer's modus operandi was in place for his next attack, which occurred August 10 at the home of Steve Boca, an Italian grocer who lived on Elysian Fields in the French Quarter. Boca discovered an attacker looming above him as he slept. The next thing he could remember, Boca was staggering from his bed with his skull fractured. As the blood flowed down his chest and back, he managed to alert his neighbor, Frank Genusa, who opened the door to discover Boca collapsing before him.

Genusa called the police and waited as Boca struggled to stay alive, losing consciousness at several points and mumbling incoherently in Italian. The grocer ended up surviving the attack but could not provide police with any description of the Axeman. Baffled detectives arrested Genusa – who had called them to the scene – in connection with the murder. He was released after a brief interrogation.

Like some other victims, Boca recalled a large figure circling him in his room before his head was split open. The attacker delivered neither threats nor explanation of any kind. The poetic nature of the Axeman's letters seemed to elude the man in real life. He entered Boca's home after removing a panel from his back door with a wooden chisel. He also used an axe found in the grocer's home and left as quickly and anonymously as he came.

The Final Victim: Mike Pepitone, Grocer in the Quarter

The saga continued some ten weeks later. Police were called to the home of an Italian grocer name Mike Pepitone on October 27, 1919. Pepitone had been beaten to death with a pipe. His wife and seven children were at home when an attacker – possibly two – went into the house and pummeled Pepitone in his bedroom. His wife said she awoke to see two men on their way out of the house. A pipe with a wing nut attached (which effectively takes the form of a metal axe) was used to kill the grocer this time. Police had no reason to suspect an axe murderer. Mrs. Pepitone gave her account to the police in a state of shock, coolly describing the events as she had seen them.

She had entered the bedroom where her husband slept after hearing noises. She found Mike on the bed with his skull cracked, his face barely recognizable, bleeding to death. In her hurry inside the bedroom she had a brush with the murderers, who slipped by her in their exit. Despite being so close to the attackers she had no detailed description. One was short; the other was tall. As the police widened the scope of the investigation, neighbors came forward and told stories of Italians paying a visit to Pepitone recently. They described two men lurking outside the store in the afternoon, at one point addressing Pepitone in Italian and having an animated discussion. It was the day before he was murdered.

CHAPTER 3: A SUSPECT LIST AS DEEP AS THE MISSISSIPPI – ON THE KILLER'S TRAIL

There was no question an Axeman was killing men, women and children in New Orleans. However, the portrayal of the murderer by police and journalists was problematic from the start. Many of the attacks attributed to the Axeman weren't perpetrated with an axe. The lead pipe used on Mike Pepitone was maybe the deadliest and most effective weapon in the spree, yet it wasn't an axe. Reporters kept this in mind for several weeks, until the Pepitone murder inexorably became an Axeman slaying. Stories referenced the latest Italian grocer who fell victim to a bloodthirsty villain who stalked the streets. The inaccuracies went unnoticed. The killer remained at large through the end of 1919 and into the following year.

Instead, the Mysterious Axman's Jazz played on and any murder victims had the potential to become one of his. If the Axeman could not find his weapon of choice following his ascent from Tartarus, who was to say he would not use a pipe or a club? If the medical reports disputed the reports of the press (as in the Laumann attack), the public managed to forget them. After all, the method was not as important as the madness. Murder was in the air.

Clues and Leads in the Maggio Killings

One challenge for detectives at the time was the compounding of murders. As soon as one investigation was launched, another murder followed. By many accounts, New Orleans was always one of the nation's murder capitals.

Detectives had few leads when they arrived at the Maggio residence in May 1918, but they did have the murder weapons: the axe and the razor. The latter, used to cut Catherine Maggio's throat, belonged to Andrew Maggio. Police haplessly arrested, held and then released the man. They started over from scratch.

A casual glance at the period reveals that axes were a standard element in New Orleans homes those days. In fact, axe murders were common for much of the early nineteenth century. One of the biggest killing sprees in American history had taken place earlier that same decade in Louisiana. A New York Times report in 1912 tallied 31 dead at the hand of an axe-murder cult known as "The Sacrifice Sect." While most of the murders were committed outside the city, several victims were claimed inside New Orleans parishes. Among them were a shopkeeper's wife and one Sacrifice Sect leader. Cult members were said to use a combination of voodoo and Christian rites in their ceremonies, and each ended in a gory axe slaying.

This bit of axman jazz played out in the countryside, in the Louisiana Rice Belt, where freed men and women worked the land under the era's Jim Crow laws. The Sacrifice Sect performed the majority of its rituals far from Black Hand extortionists and Dixieland jam bands. Reports of the Maggio family murders did recall a string of killings that were thought to be Mafia-related from the same period. Anthony Sciambra's murder, for example, became a subject of curiosity following the Maggio slaying because of the cryptic message in chalk.

"Mrs. Maggio will sit up tonight, just like Mrs. Toney," found nearby the Maggio house on the murder night, could refer to the wife of a man named Toney. As long as grocers were muscled or killed without evidence of a robbery on the premises, the connection was plausible. However, the Axeman theorists had to ignore that Tony Sciambra and his wife were shot to death (Mrs. Sciambra, for her part, wasn't targeted yet succumbed to a wound initially considered treatable – she was shot in the hip). The 1912 Sciambra attacks instead appeared connected to the brutal beatings suffered by other Italian grocers in 1910.

The Davi, Crutti and Rossetti Cases Collide

New Orleans police had their hands full throughout this period, which was dominated by Black Hand extortionists. Stores were burned, children were kidnapped, women were beaten to death and neighborhood grocers were shot or clubbed into submission, all in the interest of funding the Black Hand brigade.

This blackmailing faction of the Sicilian Mafia was known for its ruthless tactics, aimed at getting shop owners to pay protection money. Since the protection was largely symbolic, and the threats often baseless, small business owners would regularly shrug off blackmail notes. But when the Black Hand made a statement, the entire community felt the pain.

Sciambra's case reminded police of the Joseph Davi case. Davi received multiple Black Hand letters, as well as in-person solicitations, before being killed at his home (his wife, viciously hacked with a meat cleaver, survived). When police brought in suspects for questioning in the Davi killing, they asked other grocers who has been victimized to make a statement.

Two businessmen by the names of Crutti and Rossetti visited police headquarters to offer help in apprehending the same thugs who attacked them in 1910. Two Sicilian truck farmers known for their intimidation tactics were being held as suspects. They were tied to multiple beatings and considered suspects in the Davi murderers, yet no one could establish the culpability of either man.

The Web of Evidence Connects Known Mafiosi

As the cases of murder and extortion piled up throughout the period, police officials hinted at connections but continuously failed to prove a conspiracy. The similarities between the attacks on Davi, Rossetti and Crutti are considerable. Lost in the shuffle were other notable events, including the arson job at George Massachia's store on June 24, 1911. Massachia ran a grocery at the intersection of Miro and Painter Street, where he had received Black Hand letters before watching the store go up in flames.

Investigators in the Axeman case continuously scoffed at the notion Black Hand forces or rival Mafia factions were involved in any way. Citing the mob's signature use of shotguns, revolvers and dynamite, the police believed a different type of killer was on the loose. Buoyed by inaccurate reporting, mislabeled deeds and the Crescent City tendency to indulge in the fantastical, mythmaking continued to trump reality as the investigation sputtered.

The ability of a killer to stage a beating with no weapon and no evidence left on the scene could very well have represented an evolution of Black Hand enforcement techniques. The high-profile (and low return) efforts of the previous decade were ineffective. If the police could piece together an attack and small sums of money were the sole reward for long prison stretches, their jobs were a complete failure.

However, if a band of marauders wanted to make a point to victims without the public realizing the identity of the attackers, the series of raids staged between 1910 and 1920 were wildly successful. Delivering the message of blackmail in person would account for the sightings of Mafia toughs in and around the establishments of the victims prior to the slayings. In this system, no one seen could be fingered without immediate, horrifying reprisals. The racket was unimpeachable.

Earlier efforts by Black Hand figures Vito DiGiorgio and the well-traveled Joseph Monfre were not so well executed. Monfre was convicted and sentenced to twenty years in federal prison for dynamiting Carlo Graffagnino's store in 1907. Monfre was paroled years later, a fact cited by those suspecting him for the Axeman murders, yet his motives throughout the era were professional. Monfre – alternately called "Doc" Mumphrey or Mumfre in newspapers – was among the crew working the infamous Lamana kidnapping. This very ugly (and very public) case ended in the death of a young boy and life sentences for the four suspects. Monfre and his brother disappeared for several years following this grisly crime. They were never charged in connection with the murder of the Lamana boy.

For DiGiorgio's part, his role in the 1909 bombing of the Serio clothing store etched his name in New Orleans crime ledgers for good. Serio was one person willing to ignore Black Hand threats, which were possibly delivered by Monfre in his return to the New Orleans underworld. Yet DiGiorgio persevered and ended up in possession of Tony Sciambra's profitable store after the couple's 1912 murder. Neighbors of Sciambra were surprised Sciambra's brother would give up the store to another man, as it was a highly successful business. Authorities had no leads on DiGiorgio at the time of the 1914 acquisition.

DiGiorgio continued using the Sciambra store as a front for mob activities until a man named DePeche shot him and an associate in May 1916. As police took the shooter to jail, two of DiGiorgio's men opened fire on them. Both men were arrested later and after police searched their rooms, they came across weapons, bullets and numerous extortion letters, some of which were torn to pieces. The only one that wasn't destroyed was addressed to G.D. Maggio. Giuseppe (Joseph) Maggio and his wife would be the first victims of the New Orleans Axeman two years later.

Where Vito DiGiorgio Pulled the Strings

The world got considerably smaller when Vito DiGiorgio set up shop in Anthony Sciambra's store at Dauphine and Marigny. DiGiorgio completed his hostile takeover with nothing more than the acquiescence of the Sciambra family, who had to suspect he killed him. It served as a strategic location from which he could continue his ambitious underworld business without interference.

The attack by DePeche in 1916 gave him little pause, and DiGiorgio claimed he was unable to identify the shooter who killed his partner and seriously wounded him.

He was accustomed to living with pain, as a Mafia associate later confirmed, and had observed a strict code of omerta his entire life.

DePeche was not from New Orleans, leading many to believe he was an assassin from out of state, sent to move on DiGiorgio for past deeds.

The New Orleans Mafia was a complicated organization with several competing factions, but it was also a part of the nascent national syndicate.

As tribute was ordered from local mob figures, wars of independence would start if smaller bosses resisted. It was enough to make DiGiorgio plan a move to Los Angeles.

Neighbors who lived near DiGiorgio's Dauphine Street grocery saw the place as a Mafia operation through and through. Associates came and went at all hours of the day.

DiGiorgio kept out of the news until he left for L.A. in 1921, where he was the target of another assassination attempt.

DiGiorgio did survive long enough to see old New Orleans gangster associates arrive in L.A. One of them was Joseph Monfre.

CHAPTER 4: THE POLICE TACKLE THE BESUMER MURDER

Stumped by the Maggio murder, police became even more troubled trying to bring in whoever attacked Louis Besumer and Anna Lowe. When John Zanca found the couple, he called the police and saw little of his neighbors after. Zanca was questioned and released. The couple, assumed married, actually merely lived together after arriving in New Orleans three months earlier. Besumer was married and separated from his first wife. After both spent time in the hospital, Lowe became somewhat delirious and accused Besumer of murder, of spying for the Germans (it was late in WWI) and of other terrible deeds.

With World War I raging overseas, federal investigators took Lowe seriously and arrested Besumer on charges of spying against the United States of America. He was held in jail for nine months under suspicion. However, investigators failed to advance the case in any significant way. They found letters in the grocer's native Polish, but translations revealed nothing incriminating. For the second straight axe murder, the attacker used a weapon found in the victim's house, which was left at the scene of the crime. The investigation never progressed further.

Anna Lowe died in her hospital bed the following spring. No one came forward with evidence against Besumer before or after. By the time of his trial, the war had ended, nullifying any fears of his spying, if any existed. The jury acquitted him almost instantly. The date was May 1, 1919. While Besumer was in jail, three more victims were attacked. The Polish grocer was neither a spy nor the Axeman of New Orleans.

Mrs. Schneider, Sarah Laumann and a Copycat on the Scene

It is difficult to ignore the similarities in many murders attributed to the Axeman of New Orleans. In almost every case, an axe was found at the scene of the crime and many victims were Italian grocers. Robbery was never the motive, yet intimidation – and, sometimes, outright destruction – was occasionally on the agenda. For this reason detectives struggled to connect the attacks on Mrs. Edward Schneider and the young Sarah Laumann to the Axeman's other deeds. The point of entry was different in both of these attacks. The trademark chiseled-out door panel wasn't a factor. Finally, the results (though horrifying) were not fatal in either case.

Mrs. Schneider was pregnant and delivered a healthy baby two weeks later. Sarah Laumann reportedly lost teeth along with a great deal of blood as a result of her attack, but she survived. The only elements these attacks had in common with the other axe murders were the dearth of leads and the inability of investigators to examine the murder scene properly.

John D'Antonio, a retired NOPD detective who had investigated countless murders earlier that decade, told the press he believed a Dr. Jekyll & Mr. Hyde figure might be at work. D'Antonio, who'd specialized in Mafia crime, had trouble seeing how anyone could stealthily enter homes and commit the murders; how no one could name the attacker, or even describe him; and how each murder would be followed by a period of inactivity, before the attacks began again in force.

It could be anyone – a grocer, a lawyer, a pharmacist – who feels the burden of evil and suddenly seeks blood.

Romano, Cortimiglia and Boca Fall; the System Returns

Following the Schneider attack, police were as baffled as ever at the identity and methods of the Axeman. Yet the next to be struck marked a return to the original pattern. Romano was a barber, not a grocer, but he fit the

profile of a man whose business could be com-
promised. His wounds were fatal. Romano's
nieces claimed to see the killer on his way out
of their home, but their descriptions were
vague and colored by fear. They described the
intruder as remarkably light on his feet and
marveled at his ability to leave at such a fast
pace. If the same killer escaped on so many different occasions, he would have needed excep-
tional speed and grace. Romano's nieces
remarked his ability in that department other-
worldly. The investigation floundered.

In the Axeman's first attack of 1919, he
came at the world from a slightly different an-
gle. He struck in Gretna, which is right outside
of New Orleans, on the opposite banks of the
Mississippi River. Gretna had a substantial Italian population at the time. In fact, disputes
among rival political factions led to the arrest
of a suspected Black Hand crew in Gretna just
a few years earlier.

The incident in question involved Joseph
Monfre, of the Lamana kidnapping and Graf-
fagnino bombing fame. Monfre appeared in
Gretna's courthouse to respond to charges of

carrying a concealed weapon while on parole. Before Monfre's parole issues were addressed by the court it was pointed out that he was in possession of a police clerk's standard-issue gun. Monfre shrugged off this detail as a trifle while he submitted testimony without an attorney present. Monfre explained that he was delivering leaflets for an upcoming election when he was picked up by police. As for the question regarding his parole, Monfre noted he was released on the recommendation of Louisiana Governor Luther Hall. Angelo Albano and his younger brother, two mob figures, had been apprehended along with Monfre as they patrolled Gretna that night.

Clearly, the mob's grip on Gretna was as strong as it was across the river in New Orleans. The horror at the Cortimiglia house seemed to be a continuation of the murderous spree, but to a more shocking degree. While it was difficult to find a more sympathetic victim than a pregnant woman, the Axeman who killed an infant in Gretna had shattered any possible boundary that existed. Charles and Rose Cortimiglia survived this attack, and it was

Rose's testimony that put Iorlando and Frank
Jordano on trial for murder. They were both
found guilty. Iorlando's son Frank was given
the death penalty for his involvement in the killing. It appeared the Jordanos, as local grocers,
had a minor rivalry with the Cortimiglias, yet
the entire accusation was baseless. Rose re-
canted her statement the following year and
the Jordanos were released.

At this point, there seemed to be no way
the police could get a conviction in the Axeman
slayings. The investigation into Steve Boca's
murder on Elysian Fields Avenue yielded nothing. Boca was a grocer who knew nothing – or
at least would say nothing – of his assailant after the attack. His neighbor Steve Genusa had
helped get him to the hospital before he could
succumb to his injuries. Genusa was hardly considered a suspect. Boca could offer nothing of
import to the police, other than a vague description of a dark figure pummeling him in the
night. It was a refrain that played over and over
in the cases. A room or entire home was ran-
sacked or left untouched; axed victims survived
but knew nothing of the assailant; and

somewhere in the night, a fleet-footed psycho-
path danced off to safety, plotting his next attack.

After the Boca attack there were no other
murders by the Axeman of New Orleans, but
that didn't stop the public from attributing
Mike Pepitone's murder to him. Pepitone was
the victim of a brutal pipe beating. There was
no axe involved. The police watched and
waited through 1919, a year that concluded
without any grocers, young women, or Italians
falling prey to the Axeman's hand.

At least, that was the perception of law enforcement officials and the press. As for the
axe murders that continued throughout the
1920s, observers considered the connections
too circumstantial to attribute to the Axeman.
Yet New Orleans and neighboring communities
in Louisiana and the South would mourn the
deaths of many more axe murder victims in
those years. The tune to "The Mysterious Axman's Jazz" was long forgotten by then.

CHAPTER 5: THE APPARENT END TO THE MURDERS – AND A CLUE FROM CALIFORNIA

Though Pepitone's murderer used a pipe to bash in his victim's skull, his wife suggested he had an accomplice. Two men had stalked the grocer's home the previous day (according to the Times-Picayune). Then the pipe murder was attributed to the New Orleans Axeman. Some time after the eyewitness accounts stopped appearing, the crime became an axe murder. While that element of the case clearly had no basis in reality, the connections between the

Pepitone family, the New Orleans underworld and other Axeman killings are too direct to ignore.

In December 1921, the city shuddered in response to recent news from California. "Joseph Mumfre," a native of the Big Easy, had been shot dead by Esther Albano, a New Orleans woman who said she was the widow of Mike Pepitone. Mrs. Albano (formerly Mrs. Pepitone) had moved to California some time after her husband's murder and married Angelo Albano. Her new husband, of course, was a known associate of Joseph Monfre from his days on the Gretna circuit. Reports placed Albano with Monfre/Mumfre in 1916, when the two were arrested for carrying concealed weapons in the midst of their election push. Mumfre and Albano decided to become business partners in California, where they opened a grocery store. Yet their partnership soured shortly thereafter. Albano, expressing dissatisfaction with Mumfre, bought out his partner's interest in the business. Then Albano disappeared into the California night.

Where the Pepitone and Mumfre Stories Intersect

Los Angeles detectives said the woman, who claimed she was widowed – twice – by Mumfre, told them she killed the old Black Hand operator both in self-defense and in revenge. If that story held water on any level, the path of Esther Albano to California would have to be traced. She'd met Albano at a niece's wedding, she told authorities. That story turned out to be a lie. Albano and the former Mrs. Pepitone wed earlier in the year.

Why she had lived with the knowledge that Mumfre killed Mike Pepitone was also unclear. Meeting her husband's business partner would have been a jarring moment if she recognized him as her husband's killer. Meanwhile, her new husband Angelo Albano continued his business relationship with Mumfre, whether or not he knew of the connection. Was she unwilling to turn over information to the police that she felt they would not use? Was Mumfre, for his part, dogged enough to live in close communion to a woman whose husband he had killed?

Following Albano's disappearance in California, the new Mrs. Albano did bring her concerns to the police. And yet Mumfre appeared again for another shakedown of a woman he'd terrorized for several years. Mumfre calmly strolled into the Albano home and told Esther she would need to hand over protection money, while her children sat in another room. If she wanted protection, Mumfre added, she wouldn't be getting it from he husband – he would never appear in Los Angeles again. She could join him soon, or she could pay Mumfre the bill. Seeing the cards in her future, Esther Pepitone-Albano shot Mumfre on the spot.

If Joseph Mumfre (aka Doc Mumphrey) was the renowned criminal from New Orleans he was supposed to be, then Esther Albano (the former Mrs. Pepitone) had more than a small history with the man and his crew. It began in New Orleans a long time before the pipe beating, several years after the Lamana and Graffagnino cases had gripped the city's imagination.

The Deeper, Darker Past in the Big Easy

In 1910, Mike Pepitone's father Peter killed Paul DiChristina, a well-known Mafioso who had recently arrived from New York. DiChristina had made his move on Vincent Moreci, one of the top figures in the New Orleans Mafia at the time. Peter Pepitone calmly blasted DiChristina one day outside his store. In 1915, Times-Picayune reports had "Mrs. Michael Pepitone" in charge of the grocery store following Peter's trip to jail. Other Italian grocers at the time were killed, among them Anthony Sciambra (in 1912). The Sciambra death was later linked to the Axeman murders. Reporters included Sciambra – whose wife was accidentally shot as well – among the victims of an axe-carrying goon.

Yet Sciambra was certainly shot, putting his death under the category of Mafia hit. Vito DiGiorgio gained control of his profitable grocery. An attempt was then made on Moreci, though he declined to point any fingers at attackers. He resolved to settle the issue on his own. Later, another associate of DiChristina named DiMartino was shot dead. Moreci was quickly arrested and charged with the crime but found not guilty. Moreci met his end shortly after at the hands of a trio of mafia hit-men. There were witnesses on the scene, but before anyone was identified, the police arrested and held one suspect: Joseph Monfre.

DiGiorgio himself was shot in 1916, an assault he survived. Later, when Axeman murders were suggested to be Mafia retaliations, the theory was called into question because women and children were targeted by the maniac. Looking at the homicides and blackmail ploys of the Black Handers, it's safe to say there were no restrictions on the types of victims claimed.

In fact, the Mumfre rap sheet begins with a bombing of a grocer's home in 1907. Monfre, who is cited as Doc Mumphrey at times and Joseph Monfre at others (in the pre-"Mumfre" era), found himself before the parole board on several occasions. He appealed for a pardon as well as time off for good behavior. His connections within the political ranks were extensive,

as his 1916 arrest revealed. Known to be a dy-
namite-planting career criminal whose influence
extended to the governor's office, Monfre was
back on the street in 1917. In 1919, he was arrested early in the year for again carrying concealed weapons and engaging in suspicious
behavior. Yet that charge didn't stick, either.
Despite the fact that he was on parole (which
he'd just violated), Monfre was ready to return
to duty as a Mafia soldier. Any deeds attributed to the Axeman is 1918 and 1919 could
have been committed by Monfre, whether in
Gretna or the Big Easy.

In fact, Monfre was mentioned in connection
with one of the most highly publicized cases of
the era: the Lamana kidnapping. This black-
mail/ransom scheme by the local Black Hand
had gone much too far. Instead of getting their
money, the group (which included two Monfre
brothers) was urged by local Italian groups and
rival mafia factions to return the boy at once.
All parties were horrified at the events as they
unfolded. Yet someone in the group lost his
nerve and murdered the young boy, dumping
his body in a makeshift coffin by the river. Four

people went to jail for life, but the two Monfre brothers were never apprehended for their part in the crime.

Whoever was committing the murders attributed to the Axeman and Mafia, the idea that a mob-connected button man would not kill women or children had no basis in the reality of Crescent City life in 1919. Avoiding bombs and the murder of innocents became part of a code for later Mafia groups. In early twentieth-century New Orleans, no one was safe.

CHAPTER 6: FOUR NAMES, ONE CRIMINAL – THE ELUSIVE MONFRE-MUMPHREY-MUMFRE-MANFRE

Black Hand extortionists were known for their ruthlessness as well as their brazenness. From the stories – both published and circumstantial – concerning the man most often referred to as Joseph Monfre, it is obvious he was capable of committing murder on a grand scale. It was in his early days planting dynamite in the Quarter that Monfre caught the attention of Mafia higher-ups.

Worthy of protection and likely given access to the political connections of elite Mafia ringleaders, Monfre did not feel ashamed to petition for a pardon following his bombing conviction. Lawyers did the arguing for him, but Monfre was just as comfortable representing himself in court, as he cavalierly did upon a trip back to jail for carrying weapons in Gretna while still on parole.

The sensational testimony that came out of Monfre's mouth the day of his court appearance stunned reporters on the scene, but told an even bigger story – Monfre was neither intimidated by law enforcement nor worried about serving long stretches in prison. He had done more than seven years on the dynamiting conviction, yet was arrested with concealed weapons at least twice on parole.

Monfre told the court at one parole hearing that his lawyer lost interest in the case, because there were no witnesses, and that the state was sure to lose. Therefore, he hadn't shown up, confident that Monfre would acquit himself well before the court. He continued that he wasn't paying the attorney since he was canvassing for his chosen Gretna politician – Monfre's excuse for why the opposing (incumbent) party had sent him back to jail. Of course, noting that he was released on Governor Hall's recommendation, there was little reason to suspect he'd be locked up for long. Court reporters weren't used to hearing accounts of this nature. They rushed back to their newspaper offices to file the story.

Yet Monfre continued his activities, eluding even the reporters who covered the city's web of organized crime on a daily basis. Only one report of the era managed to connect the name Joseph Monfre to "Doc Mumphrey," a man said to run a pharmacy in between stints in local and federal prison. By the time the wife of Mike Pepitone shot down a New Orleans thug and fingered him as the Axeman, his name was Mumfre. The California certificate of death listed him as Manfre.

Monfre was in and out of jail during the mid-1910s, but he returned to the scene in 1917, as the Black Hand's influence on the French Quarter was in decline. Prohibition and its special brand of spoils lay ahead, but the old-school operators still knew how to extort cash from the smaller men on the block. Monfre – in all his different aliases – had no qualms about dropping the hammer to make money and please Mafioso bosses in turn.

The Strings Mafiosi Played Inside the Pen and Out

Reports from the era tell the tale of a crime ring backed by aggressive lawyers and supportive of political causes. In return for a guaranteed voting bloc, politicians were open to returning favors to their Mafia supporters. Monfre, however brazenly, referenced this point during his court date. Articles from years earlier recounted a brawl inside the local jail when Monfre's attorney wasn't granted access to his client. Other newspaper references to casual shootouts between known Mafia strongmen reflect a calm acceptance between the police and their perceived targets. Some disputes were clearly better off in the hands of the rival Mafia factions.

Detective D'Antonio, whose opinion of the Axeman identity caused a stir, filed reports throughout the era as the chief inspector in many Mafia-suspected crimes. Fluent in Italian and known throughout the parishes as the police liaison to the community, D'Antonio was the bridge between Crescent City Cosa Nostra and the establishment. He was the man ostensibly assigned to subdue the Mafia through his knowledge of the language and the subtleties of the culture.

D'Antonio is mentioned most often in cases where the killer remains at large, or when the killer pulled off a daring escape. Assigned to mob hits and shakedowns on a regular basis, it is likely D'Antonio was assigned some of the toughest murders of the era, including several of the early killings (ca. 1910) later attributed to the New Orleans Axeman. Yet a murder he was certainly not assigned to investigate – the Joseph Romano killing – brought him out of retirement to divulge his theories to the world. D'Antonio hypothesized the city had a modern Jekyll and Hyde on its hands, a man who could be anything – a pharmacist, perhaps – at one moment and a bloodthirsty killer the next.

D'Antonio was also vocal about his belief that the killer was unlikely to have anything to do with the Mafia. It didn't matter that small Italian grocers were receiving threats from intimidating men just before the attacks; or that the victims were the clear targets of Black Handers; or that purported Axeman slayings were likely mob retaliation hits. Though all these factors would have pushed modern investigators to precisely that conclusion, D'Antonio believed in a killer who could change personalities and stalk the night after leaving imaginative letters for newspaper editors. Of course, if they weren't Mafia-related, and the murders he tracked from 1910-1912 were also the Axeman's doing, then his record on the police force would have been unimpeachable.

In D'Antonio's time, the highest officer of the New Orleans Police Department met his end at the hand of Mafia assassins. In one of the most explosive moments in the city's history, Mafia henchmen gunned down Chief of Police David Hennessey in front of his home in 1890. Local residents, fed up with the growing influence of organized crime among Sicilian immigrants, took matters into their own hands and lynched Italian prisoners held in county jails. The stakes were high for criminal and law enforcement officials alike during this time, especially when the public got wind of the inner workings of the justice and enforcement divisions.

D'Antonio's speculations meant little at the time to police and public alike. They put on official record that the mob was not involved; that the killer from his time was still terrorizing the city; and that no one could catch him. Afterwards, he kept his theories to himself as the killer continued on the lam. Any insider at police headquarters in 1918 could swear to one thing without hesitation: it would have been impossible for Detective D'Antonio to be unaware of the identity of Joseph Monfre of New Orleans.

CHAPTER 7: OMERTA IN THE BIG EASY – HOW A VOW OF SILENCE KEPT KILLERS IN THE SHADOWS

Throughout the investigation of Black Hand killings, Axeman slayings and everything in between, the reluctance of Italian eyewitnesses to come forward with information hindered the judicial process at every level. In the early manifestations of feuding Mafia factions it was clear that the parties had plans of their own for leveling justice. Yet innocent victims later showed a blatant unwillingness to cooperate with the New Orleans police.

There were occasional exceptions. An issue outside the Peter Pepitone grocery in 1915 caused reports to be filed by a woman living alone in the Quarter. Her husband had killed Paul DiChristina, yet was hiding out upon his release (just a few years later) from federal prison. In many ways, it appeared Peter Pepitone was creating another alibi for himself. Using his wife as bait, he sent word to the police that he was playing by the rules. If he had to take down another Mafia strongman, he would do so. After the killing of DiChristina's, a bona fide Mafia kingpin, the grudge against Pepitone would not be dropped until the rival family was satisfied. That battle would come.

Victims of the men alleged to have attacked the Joseph Davi family in 1910 also came forward at the request of police, but that landmark murder had stunned the community for the killer's brutal attack on Mrs. Davi. Hacking at the woman with a meat cleaver, the assailant finished off Davi while his wife lay dying on the floor. Local Italians were horrified at the assault, sending a normally reticent group toward the police with at least the appearance of cooperation.

Nonetheless, they didn't finger anyone the police were holding, whether they had no evidence or they didn't want to say anything. The power of omerta – the Sicilian code of silence – held sway over most internal disputes in the community. Police found that murders followed murders, rather than investigations following murders. In a thorny world of organized crime, informers are the detective's lifeblood. Yet in the Italian-dominated Quarter, murders constantly went unsolved.

The Final Showdown: Where Omerta Failed and Order Was Restored

In a world that often appears savage, the American Mafia had a variety of codes that were meant to maintain a level of decency in the community. Allegiance to the family trumped all concerns, but mistakes – both moral and professional – could break the family bonds in an instant. Mafia wives were to be respected, as were the women and children of the world; murders would need to be approved or risk bloody reprisal; and in no circumstances was the code of omerta to be broken.

In the case of the long-cherished code of silence, it is easy to see where the system failed in New Orleans. Following the shocking lynchings of 1890, the steady stream of Italians arriving to the Crescent City made them an essential part of the community. It was impossible to ignore 80% of the Latin Quarter, and the acceptance continued as Catholic rituals were shared with the residents of French ancestry.

Yet Italians after the turn of the century began to fear fellow Italians. When your children were no longer safe (no matter how young and innocent), when anyone walking to the corner grocer for bread could become a victim of an explosion, when wives were hit in the crossfire, the rules became meaningless.

Esther Pepitone stared investigators in the face in October 1919 and told them she didn't see anything other than two men on their way out of her home. She said one was of taller stature and one was shorter. The police consumed this insignificant piece of evidence and embarked on another unsuccessful investigation. The murder of Mike Pepitone was never solved, Axeman or not.

Esther Pepitone has probably seen Joseph Mumfre around the time Vincent Moreci was shot. Her grocery store had been on the minds of local thugs even since her father-in-law killed Paul DiChristina. Her nephew and sons had been planning to face the revenge of the family for years. Yet Esther took them with her to Los Angles and married the man who was closest to their father's killer. Albano knew of Mumfre's legacy firsthand and married her regardless.

Yet the code broke down when Joseph Monfre led Angelo Albano to his death in California. Esther waited patiently for him to arrive home, but it was clear that day would never come. She finally left omerta twisting in the wind while she told police she wanted his murder investigated. Vito DiGiorgio by then had established himself as one of the biggest gangsters in town. His old friend Joseph Monfre came to appreciate his connections.

No matter what Esther Albano told the police, they wouldn't pursue the man she believed killed her two husbands. Then every aspect of the Mafia code evaporated when Monfre approached the Albano home in December 1921.

Vito DiGiorgio had decamped to New Orleans following another shootout with Mafia gunmen. The bullet wounds in DiGiorgio's legs and chest forced him into a semi-permanent grimace. He returned to New Orleans while he plotted his next moves in the changing times of Prohibition. That left Joseph Monfre to his own devices.

Unfortunately for the old Black Hander, Esther Pepitone-Albano had decided her days of acquiescence had ended. Monfre showed up and calmly asked, as a matter of courtesy to a friend of the family (and a business partner to Angelo), if Esther wouldn't have a word with him in the adjoining room. Esther replied that he could join her in her bedroom, where loaded guns sat in her dresser drawer.

Their conversation developed along the lines that were typical for Monfre since his days of rigging stores with dynamite. She could give him a little money to stay away from her home for the time being, or he would begin to think of ways to make her life miserable. Monfre's manner was nonchalant. He puffed on a cigarette and smiled as Esther dabbed at her forehead with a handkerchief. She moved to the dresser. Monfre smiled again and mentioned that maybe she'd see Angelo Albano again if she paid. In fact, maybe the seven children downstairs would grow up to be healthy adults. She could watch them get married and have children of their own. She would become a grandmother and see an entire generation blossom around her. Los Angeles would be beautiful in ways New Orleans was not.

Somewhere during the speech, Esther Albano noted where Monfre had placed the gun on his person. She could see the bulge in his left breast beneath the suit jacket. She turned to the mirror and dabbed at her forehead once again. She told Monfre she would have to see how much money she had. Angelo's done well, Monfre replied. Esther Albano went into the dresser for money and pulled out a loaded revolver. She shot Monfre with every bullet in the gun.

Her children came running from downstairs and found the man who had killed their father and stepfather bleeding to death in front of them. Esther Albano told them to call the police. Then she sat down on the bed. Breaking the code had been as pointless as following the code. The nights passed the same, code or not. She barely mourned Mike Pepitone, a petty and violent man whose insolence was typical of the entire family. They would fight their wars themselves, Mile told her, without help from any crooked New Orleans cops. They were only in it for the money, he said – even D'Antonio, who let them kill the Italians in 1890.

If there were any disputes from here on out, he said, they would be fought by the Pepitones in the interest of the family, and their honor. DiChristina came a long way to intimidate Peter Pepitone and went to the morgue for his troubles. Mike was just as dismissive when the thugs came in 1919 – not for blood, but for money. It would never be enough. Mike told them, so he was ready to fight.

But Mike lost his war. Peter Pepitone, in hiding across the river, had lost his war. Angelo Albano had lost his war, too. When Esther Pepitone killed Monfre, she won.

While One Killer Exits, Others Fade Away

New Orleans detectives liked the idea of a cut-and-dried package, complete with a bow tied across the top. Joseph Mumfre, in all his formulations, terrorized the city for nearly a decade. Now he had been shot dead by a New Orleans woman, one who felt the sting of his deeds firsthand. Monfre's movements in and out of jail would be traced to reveal he could have committed every Axeman murder committed during those years.

The Axeman of New Orleans was dead. The city celebrated. Somewhere, in the darkest corners of the city's most squalid parish, a man whistled "The Mysterious Axman's Jazz" and grinned. He would never be caught.

BIBLIOGRAPHY

New Orleans Times-Picayune Historical Archive

New York Times Archive

Mike Dash blog: http://aforteantinthear-chives.wordpress.com/2009/07/10/fresh-light-on-the-axeman-of-new-orleans/

Cold Cases: Famous Unsolved Mysteries, Crimes, and Disappearances in America by Hel-ena Katz
Serial Killers and Media Circuses by Dirk Gib-son

"DiGiorgio: The First Crime Boss of Los Ange-les?" by Richard N. Warner. The Informer, Vol. 3, No. 3, July 2010.

READY FOR MORE?

We hope you enjoyed reading this series. If you are ready to read similar stories, check out other books in the *Cold Case Crimes* series:

Jeff Davis 8: The True Story Behind the Unsolved Murder That Allegedly Inspired True Detective, Season One (By Fergus Mason)

Jefferson Davis Parish has been described as quaint, and in many ways it certainly is. For anyone from a big city much of the area, especially out among the farms, is like a trip in a time machine. For a sleepy rural community, however, Jefferson Davis is a lot more violent than you'd expect, and these days cheap, potent rocks of cocaine are at the root of a lot of that violence.

Crack addicts are famously willing to do just

about anything to subsidize their habit so street prostitution has become a real issue, mostly concentrated in the town's poorer neighborhoods south of the railway track. Prostitution – especially on the street – is a dangerous business, so the sheriff's office weren't too surprised when the first one turned up dead. As the body count climbed people started to take notice, but despite all their efforts the killings continued until eight women were dead.

This book traces one of the most fascinating unsolved crimes in the history of Louisiana. In 2014, many believe it became one of the inspirations for the first season of HBO's "True Detective." But the crimes in this book are much more shocking than anything captured on TV.

The Martyr of El Salvador: The Assassination of Óscar Romero (By Reagan Martin)

Óscar Romero, a respected Catholic priest, called on soldiers, as Christians, to put down their arms and stop carrying out the governments order to strip citizens of the most basic human rights...for this he was assassinated. For over 30 years, his murder has gone unsolved.

Who would murder a priest who only wanted to stop the injustice? And more importantly, why is it that, with substantial evidence naming the murderers involved, was nothing done to convict those guilty of murdering the country's beloved archbishop?

Annihilation In Austin: The Servant Girl Annihilator Murders of 1885 (By Tim Huddleston)

Murder. Chaos. Outrage. This was the mode in Texas' capital city, Austin from 1884 to 1885. The city had been haunted by a string of bloody murders. Women were not just killed-- they were dragged alive from their beds, taken outside where they were often tortured and then murdered. Six of the victims, all women, were found dead with sharp objects inserted in their ears.

As horrifying as the murders were, what's more horrifying is that the person who committed these heinous acts of violence was never found. To this day it remains one of the most famous unsolved crimes. It has long been suspected by several noted historians that the real killer may have been none other than Jack the Ripper.

Written with gripping, page turning suspense, this book brings you back in time to Austin, Texas, so you can experience the horror and panic for yourself. Faint at heart turn away!

The Galapagos Murder: The Murder Mystery That Rocked the Equator (By Fergus Mason)

The Galapagos Islands are a scientist's haven. Home to rare creatures, it was made famous by Charles Darwin and is the ideal spot for study, relaxation...and murder?

In September 1929 two settlers arrived on the desolate island of Floreana. They dreamed of escaping it all and were living the dream, until an arrogant Baroness and her lovers arrived. Turning an island paradise into a living hell, the Baroness suddenly disappeared without a trace. To this day, no one is sure what happened to her.

This is the story of love, paradise, betrayal, and murder. It will have you thinking twice before you ever yearn to escape to your own tropical paradise!

Young, Queer, and Dead: A Biography of San Francisco's Most Overlooked Serial Killer, The Doodler (By Reagan Martin)

The Zodiac Killer may have been San Francisco's most notorious serial killer, but another equally cruel killer was also stalking the streets at the same time, and, just like the Zodiac Killer, has never been arrested for his crimes. The difference is, while the Zodiac Killer's murder spree was heavily publicized, this other killer, nicknamed The Doodler, went unreported by the media and is nearly unknown today.

How did this ruthless killer become almost forgotten? Because he didn't target helpless women or children--he targeted gays--and in the 70s many people believed they had it coming; if they would just stop being gay, then all would be well.

In this gripping short book, you will go on the trail for one of the most brutal killers who ever lived. Read about why his victims were disregarded by a homophobic press, and how he was positively identified by three escaped victims...only to walk away free without being arrested.

Getting Away With Murder: 15 Chilling Cold Cases That Will Make You Think Twice About Going Outside (By William Webb)

Despite a decline in the number of murders in the United States since the 1960s, thousands go unsolved each year. As of 2013, the solve rate was at an all time low at only 65 percent of the total committed.

The 15 murders profiled in this book were committed between 1958 and 2014. The oldest of the set involves the bizarre murder of Pearl Eaton, one of the famous Ziegfeld Follies Girls of the 1920s. From the beginning, the crime had no leads or suspects and remains among the coldest of the 15 unsolved crimes. The most recent – the murder of four members of the McStay family found buried in the California desert in November 2013 – is under active investigation.

NEWSLETTER OFFER

Don't forget to sign up for your newsletter to grab your free book:

http://www.absolutecrime.com/newsletter